WORLD IN CRISIS

THE RACE TO END
EPIDEMICS

Robyn Hardyman

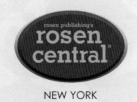

rosen publishing's
rosen
central®

NEW YORK

Published in 2015 by The Rosen Publishing Group, Inc.
29 East 21st Street
New York, NY 10010

Produced for Rosen by Calcium Creative Ltd.
Editor for Calcium Creative Ltd.: Sarah Eason
Designer: Paul Myerscough
Photo research: Rachel Blount

Library of Congress Cataloging-in-Publication Data

Hardyman, Robyn, author.
The race to end epidemics/by Robyn Hardyman.—First edition.
     pages cm.—(World in crisis)
Includes bibliographical references and index.
ISBN 978-1-4777-7840-1 (library bound)
1. Epidemics—Juvenile literature. 2. Communicable diseases—Juvenile literature. I. Title.
RA653.5.H37 2015
614.4—dc23

                                                        2013051263

Manufactured in Malaysia

Photo credits: Cover: Istockimage: Pressmaster; Inside: Dreamstime: Johnathan Andrews 19, Antonella865 22, Abhijith Ar 6, Arindam Banerjee 9, Beaniebeagle 37, Djembe 12, 31, Fmua 30, Henrikhl 40, Lisavan 5, Alexandr Mitiuc 14, Samrat35 23, Vladvitek 4; Shutterstock: Africa924 42, 43, Angellodeco 45, ArchMan 38, Asianet-Pakistan 32, Hagit Berkovich 34, Caimacanul 35, Andrea Danti 39, Tomas Fritz 20, Frontpage 28, Frances L Fruit 13, Jose Gil 27, Hinochika 11, Luiscar74 33, Martynowi.cz 16, Vucicevic Milos 26, Monkey Business Images 25, Mrfiza 41, Pieter 21, Posztos 17, Santibhavank P 18, Spirit of America 24, 44, Stanislaw Albert H. Teich 29, Tokarski 10, TonyV3112 8, ShaunWilkinson 36; Wikimedia Commons: Jeffrey Gluck 15, James le Palmer 7.

Contents

What Is an Epidemic?

Disease has always been a threat to humankind. It has often shaped history, forcing populations to move or wiping out entire communities. Some diseases, such as cancer, are a huge danger to human health but cannot be passed from person to another. The diseases that can be passed between people, such as malaria and tuberculosis, are called infectious diseases—and they cause epidemics.

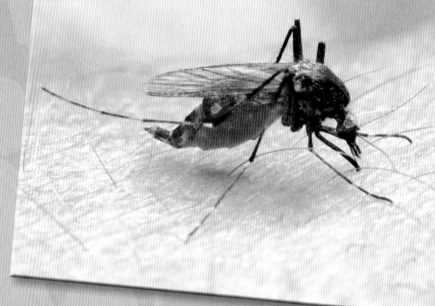

Malaria is carried by a type of mosquito. Humans catch the disease when the mosquitoes bite them. Malaria is one of the most widespread infectious diseases in the world today.

Large-scale Infection

An epidemic is not a disease. It is an event. When an infectious disease occurs on a large scale, it is called an epidemic. This means that the disease infects more people, over a wider area, and for a longer period than is normal. Any infectious disease can cause an epidemic, but there are some that occur more often than others around the world, and are a bigger threat to human life. When a disease is present in a country's population all the time it is said to be endemic. Malaria, for example, is endemic in some tropical areas of Africa, Asia, and South America.

The Challenge

Despite all the medical knowledge we have today, the impact of epidemics around the world is huge. Known infectious diseases can be hard to prevent and treat. They spread quickly and may become resistant to drug treatments. Furthermore, new strains, or types, of disease are constantly emerging. Some arise from our animal populations, while others are new versions of diseases we already know about. Scientists and health workers all over the world are trying to keep pace with epidemics, to combat their threats.

The Cost

Epidemics are the major cause of death in the less developed countries of the world. The social cost is high because communities are devastated by disease. Parents die, leaving children orphaned and in need of care until they reach adulthood.

Epidemics have immense economic costs, too. People who are unwell, or who die, cannot work and contribute to their country's economy. In a poor country, this can seriously affect people's hopes of raising themselves out of poverty. Also, the cost of the work carried out to prevent and treat epidemic diseases is enormous—billions of dollars are spent every year fighting them.

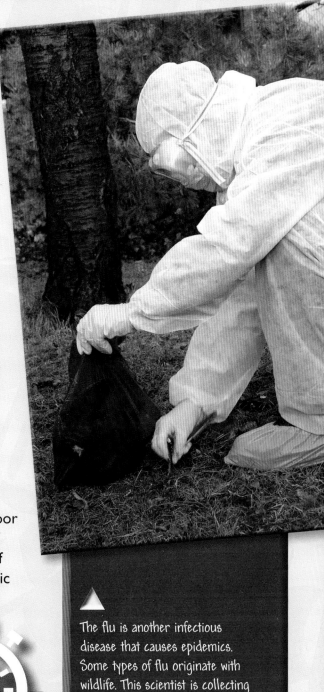

The flu is another infectious disease that causes epidemics. Some types of flu originate with wildlife. This scientist is collecting a bird to examine it for bird flu.

COUNTDOWN!

The World Health Organization (WHO) estimates that there are about 9 million cases of tuberculosis each year, and 219 million cases of malaria. These are just two of the diseases that cause epidemics.

CHAPTER ONE

How Epidemics Happen

Thanks to modern science we have come to better understand how epidemics occur. In the past, people often thought disease on a huge scale was a punishment sent from God for their sins. Now that our understanding of the science behind epidemics is improving, we can work more effectively to control them.

Infectious Disease Takes Hold

When microorganisms called pathogens invade the body, they cause disease. The three main types of pathogen are viruses, bacteria, and protozoa, and they can be carried through the air, by animals, or in water. Viruses are the smallest microorganisms, but they can be the deadliest. They invade living cells and force them to make many copies of the virus. These then break out of the host cells and invade more cells. Viruses cause some

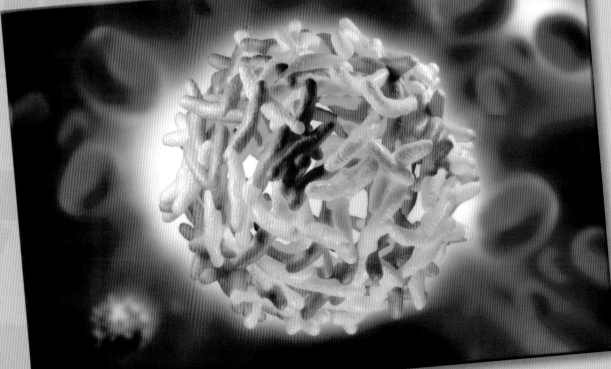

This is an illustration of the virus that causes yellow fever. The disease is spread by mosquitoes. Although yellow fever can be mild, if left untreated it can also be fatal.

of the worst epidemic diseases, such as Acquired Immunodeficiency Syndrome (AIDS), measles, and influenza, better known as "the flu."

Bacteria are all around us, and inside us. Most are harmless, and some even help us, such as the bacteria in our digestive system. However, once disease-causing bacteria enter the body they can reproduce very quickly. They produce poisons that damage cells or affect body processes. Bacteria cause diseases such as cholera and tuberculosis.

Protozoa are single-celled organisms, like bacteria, but larger and often spread by insects. They cause diseases such as malaria and sleeping sickness.

Disease Out of Control

The extent of disease in a population can reach epidemic level for several reasons. If a new disease arises, people have no resistance to that disease, and so it spreads quickly from one person to another. General poor health in a population, as a result of famine or poor living conditions, will cause low resistance to disease. Epidemics also begin when the food or water supply becomes infected, which can be the result of pollution, a natural disaster, or war. Many people then become infected at one time.

LOOK TO THE PAST

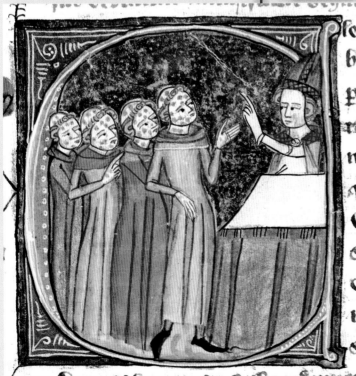

One of the most deadly epidemics in history was the bubonic plague, or Black Death, in the mid-fourteenth century. This plague, carried by fleas living on black rats, originated in central Asia and traveled along trade routes to Europe, where it killed at least 50 million people in just four years. It took 150 years for the population of Europe to recover from this devastating blow.

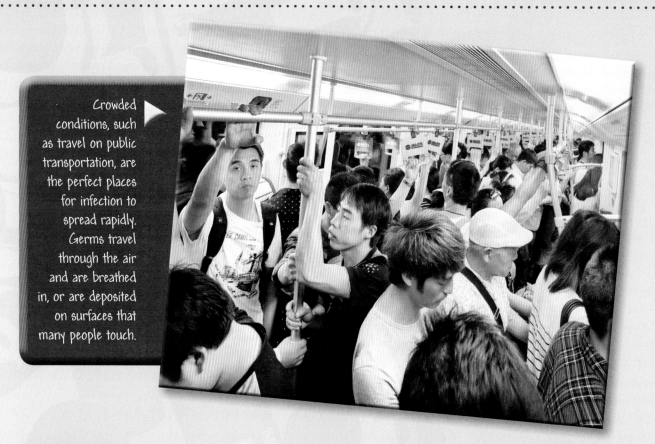

Crowded conditions, such as travel on public transportation, are the perfect places for infection to spread rapidly. Germs travel through the air and are breathed in, or are deposited on surfaces that many people touch.

Spreading Like Wildfire

The countries worst hit by epidemics most often are in the developing world. People in the poorest countries have the lowest resistance to disease, the greatest exposure to sources of infection, and the least developed health systems. In this age of mass global travel, however, a disease that originates in developing countries can quickly spread around the world.

The Disease Carriers

Insects often spread infectious diseases. Mosquitoes, for example, carry malaria, yellow fever, and dengue fever. They breed in water, and bite people living and working nearby. Some mosquitoes live in places where they mostly feed on animals, but when conditions change, they can transfer to humans. For example, monkeys that live high up in the rainforest canopy are frequently bitten by mosquitoes carrying the yellow fever virus. When people enter rainforests, the mosquitoes come into contact with humans and bite them as well. Yellow fever then spreads through the human population.

Diseases such as influenza are spread more easily. The flu virus travels through the air in water droplets when people cough and sneeze. It can also lie on everyday surfaces that people touch. In our overcrowded cities, the disease can spread through the population like wildfire. If the strain of flu is new and our resistance to it is low, we are less likely to recover before we have passed the disease on to others.

Infection can also spread through water and food. If a water supply becomes infected with cholera bacteria, for example, everyone who uses that water will get sick. This often happens after a natural disaster, when a clean water supply is unavailable. Food can also be infected by bacteria, such as *E-coli,* making people sick when they eat it.

Transporting the Problem

Today, an outbreak of infection in one part of the world, such as Beijing, China, can quickly lead to an outbreak in another part of the world, such as New York City. People travel by air all the time, carrying infections with them and passing them to others. We import our food from all over the world, and that, too, can become contaminated.

Epidemic Cycle

Epidemics have a beginning and an end. Some are seasonal, such as influenza, which spreads more easily in colder weather, when people's resistance is lowered. Malaria mosquitoes are inactive in cold weather, so the disease is less common in cooler places. Gradually, people build up a resistance to infections, too. As more people are treated, the disease finds fewer hosts to attack, and eventually dies out.

Temporary shelters set up after the 2010 earthquake in Haiti. Diseases can easily reach epidemic levels in crowded conditions such as these.

Pandemics

Epidemics can break out anywhere in the world. When a disease spreads to more than one continent, and affects a vast number of people, it becomes a pandemic. A pandemic brings entirely new challenges of treatment and control.

When a Pandemic Happens

Pandemics occur when diseases are strong enough to resist the body's natural defenses and are carried quickly around the world by people and goods. Pandemics are more serious than epidemics because more people get sick. The human immune system normally recognizes pathogens that attack the body. It produces substances called antibodies to destroy them. An epidemic occurs when the disease presents more of a challenge to the immune system and we cannot quickly fight it off with antibodies. In a pandemic, so many people become infected, and cannot fight off the disease quickly, that it has time to spread to even more people. Some of those people then travel to other areas, taking the disease with them—and the process of infection continues in the new locations.

Modern forms of transport, such as air travel, have made the threat of disease spreading, and therefore pandemics, greater than ever before.

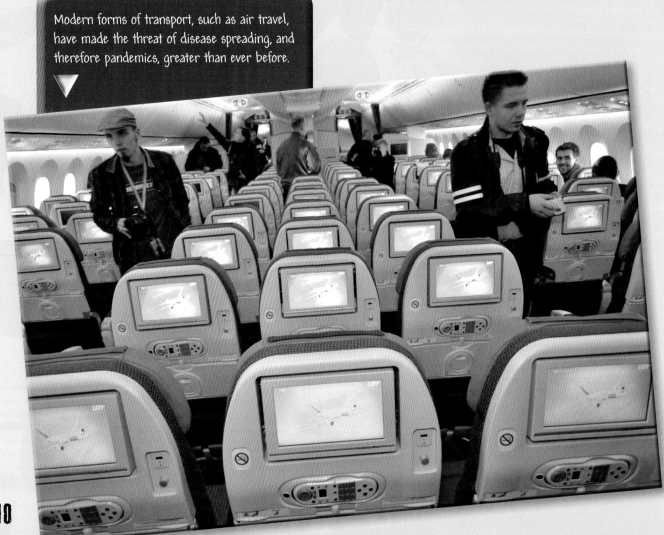

When a pandemic hits, the authorities must act quickly to contain the outbreak. Public health education and control measures, such as minimizing public events, are essential. Doctors and hospitals prepare for increased levels of patients and admissions. Drug companies work quickly to produce drugs to prevent and treat the disease.

A Constant Threat

In recent years most of the worldwide disease scares, such as bird flu and severe acute respiratory syndrome (SARS), have not developed into full pandemics. History teaches us, however, always to be on guard. On June 11, 2009, the WHO announced that the continuing outbreak of Influenza A/H1N1, or "swine flu," was officially a pandemic—the first of the twenty-first century.

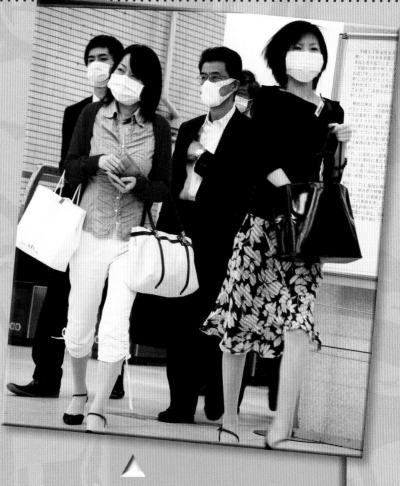

When an epidemic or pandemic occurs, people try to protect themselves from infection by wearing face masks. There is no proof, however, that masks give any effective protection to the wearer.

LOOK TO THE PAST

One of the worst pandemics in modern history was the flu pandemic of 1918–1920. As World War I drew to a close, a virus swept the whole world, affecting about one-fifth of the global population. It targeted young adults especially, up to the age of about 40. This was a new strain of flu, and nobody was immune to it. Estimates say that more than 50 million people died—a greater number than those killed during the four years of the war itself.

CHAPTER TWO

Epidemics Today

There are a number of diseases in the world today that create epidemics. Some of them are mostly confined to the developing world. Others can spread anywhere. Together, these diseases pose the biggest challenge to global health.

Where Disease Strikes

The developed countries of the world suffer less from epidemics than developing countries. Advances in science and technology have helped to eradicate some of the worst diseases from the developed world, and improved living conditions and health care keep outbreaks of disease under control. Also, some of the conditions that allow disease to take hold, such as extreme climate changes and poor animal welfare, are not as big a problem in the developed world. In the developing world, conditions often lead to uncontrollable disease outbreaks. The limited health care systems in these countries also struggle to cope with outbreaks of disease when they occur.

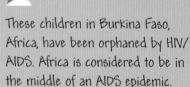

These children in Burkina Faso, Africa, have been orphaned by HIV/AIDS. Africa is considered to be in the middle of an AIDS epidemic.

There are still plenty of diseases, however, that can spread anywhere in the world, creating an epidemic or a pandemic. Every year, people everywhere are also threatened with new strains of the flu, and the HIV/AIDS pandemic affects rich and poor alike in developed and developing countries.

A Different Kind of Epidemic

While, strictly speaking, an epidemic involves an infectious disease, health professionals today talk of another major "epidemic" that is challenging many developed countries. This is obesity. An alarming number of people in the United States, for example, are seriously overweight. Many Americans are eating too much, and eating the wrong foods.

Many lead inactive lifestyles, as well. This creates major health problems for obese individuals, such as heart disease and diabetes. The consequences for the future health of the population are just as serious as those posed by a flu epidemic. For the first time in history, experts are saying that the life expectancy of currently obese generations may be lower than that of their parents and grandparents.

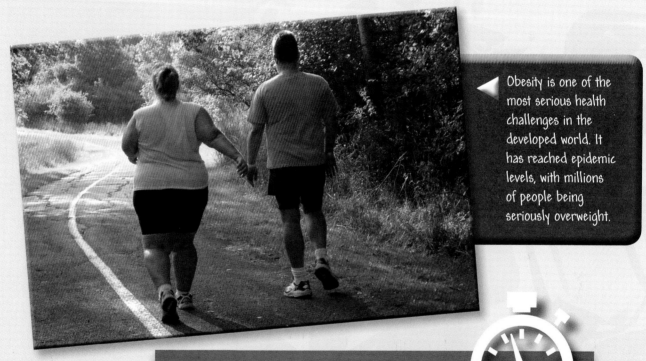

Obesity is one of the most serious health challenges in the developed world. It has reached epidemic levels, with millions of people being seriously overweight.

COUNTDOWN!

The Centers for Disease Control and Prevention (CDC) in the United States has developed a Pandemic Severity Index for influenza. This has five categories of increasing seriousness. For each category, the CDC estimates the number of likely deaths from the disease, as a number of people and as a percentage of those infected. This helps communities prepare and plan for an epidemic or a pandemic.

Malaria

Malaria is one of the major causes of illness around the world, leading to about 800,000 deaths each year. This terrible disease usually has its worst impact among children. Malaria exists in many areas of the world where the climate is warm and humid. This tends to be the tropics, in Asia, the Americas, and Africa.

Malaria is not strictly experienced as an epidemic, because in the parts of the world where it occurs most, the disease is permanently present, or endemic. It never goes away, unlike the flu or cholera. However, because of its severity, scientists are targeting malaria in their race to control the spread of infectious diseases worldwide.

How Malaria Takes Hold

Malaria is spread by the bite of a female from a type of mosquito called *Anopheles*. The insect breeds in warm, still water and multiplies rapidly. The mosquito's saliva contains protozoa called plasmodiums, which enter a person's blood when he or she is bitten, leading to infection. Plasmodiums travel to the liver, where they reproduce then burst back into the blood vessels, causing fever. The most serious kind of malaria is caused by *Plasmodium falciparum*. It has to be treated differently from the other most common kind of malaria, caused by *Plasmodium vivax*.

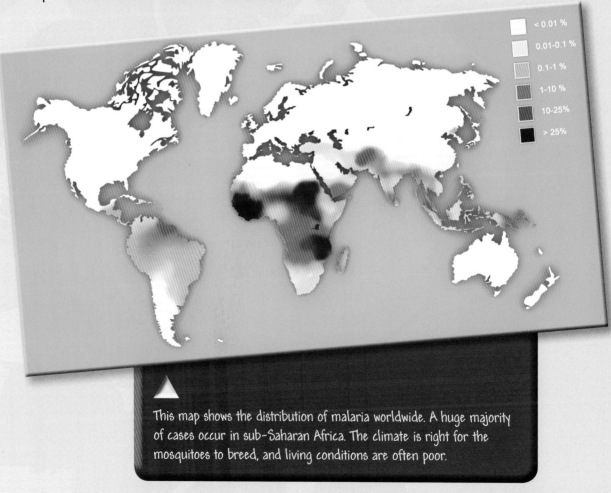

	< 0.01 %
	0.01-0.1 %
	0.1-1 %
	1-10 %
	10-25%
	> 25%

This map shows the distribution of malaria worldwide. A huge majority of cases occur in sub-Saharan Africa. The climate is right for the mosquitoes to breed, and living conditions are often poor.

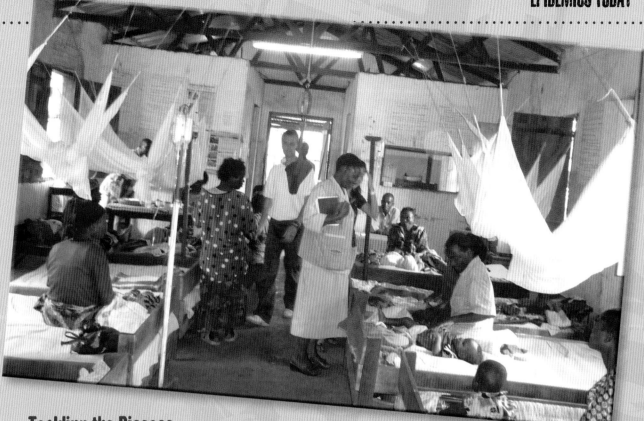

Tackling the Disease

After a mosquito has bitten a person, the symptoms of malaria can take up to one month to begin. Malaria causes fever, and weakness, vomiting, and fits, and sometimes difficulty with breathing. Without treatment, patients often die, especially if they are children. The illness can, however, be treated with drugs called antibiotics, which, if taken for just a few days, can save a child's life. In many African countries, however, small and remote village communities have little or no health care. Parents often walk for days with a sick child to find treatment. If the disease has had time to take a strong hold, that child may not survive.

Over time, plasmodiums can build up a resistance to the drugs most commonly used against them, which is why the key to defeating this terrible disease lies in prevention. Taking just a few simple steps to prevent people catching the disease can have a dramatic effect on controlling it.

These children with malaria are being treated in a clinic in Tanzania, Africa. Clinics like this one are always very busy.

COUNTDOWN!

Somewhere in the world, a child dies every minute from malaria. According to WHO, about 3.3 billion people—half the world's population —are at risk of catching the disease.

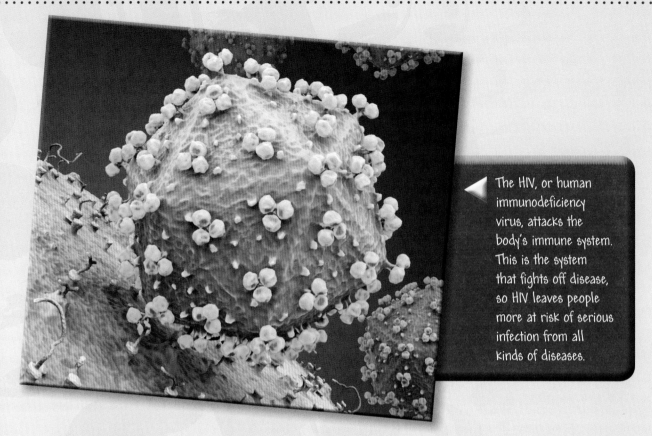

The HIV, or human immunodeficiency virus, attacks the body's immune system. This is the system that fights off disease, so HIV leaves people more at risk of serious infection from all kinds of diseases.

HIV and AIDS

In the early 1980s, doctors were mystified by a new condition that seemed to appear with no obvious cause. Patients became ill with diseases that were not usually serious, but the immune system in their bodies could not fight them off and they died. This condition was acquired immunodeficiency syndrome (AIDS), and it spread rapidly. By 1990, the disease had affected people throughout the world.

What Causes AIDS?

Scientists soon found that the cause of AIDS is a virus. The human immunodeficiency virus attacks the immune system, leaving patients vulnerable to all kinds of infection, including the serious lung condition pneumonia. The virus can lie dormant, or inactive, in the body for a long time, so that people with HIV are not always sick. About 40 million people are living with HIV today, including more than 3 million children.

HIV is passed from one person to another via body fluids, through sexual contact, blood transfusions, or from a mother to her unborn baby. Everyday contact with an infected person does not spread the disease. Many people live for years without knowing they are infected. It is only when AIDS develops that they realize they are very sick.

African Tragedy

Although HIV and AIDS exist around the world, most sufferers live in the developing world, especially in Africa. In the worst affected countries, more than one in five people aged 15 to 49 carry the virus.

Most have caught HIV from unprotected sex or from their mothers before, at, or after birth. Millions of African children have lost both their parents to AIDS, or have parents who are too sick to care for them.

Fighting HIV

There are drugs available to treat people who have HIV. The drugs cannot cure the disease, but they can stop the disease from moving forward, and so prevent people from developing AIDS. This is effective in the developed world. However, in the poorest countries these drugs are too expensive for many people to buy, even though drug companies have agreed to reduce their cost. People also have poor access to the drugs because their health care systems are limited.

SCIENCE SOLUTIONS

HIV Virus

Many scientists around the world are working to find a vaccine to protect people against HIV. A vaccine, which helps provide immunity to a disease, would be the best way to defeat HIV, but it is proving difficult to achieve, because the virus is so complex.

HIV sufferers take many drugs every day to keep them from developing AIDS.

▽

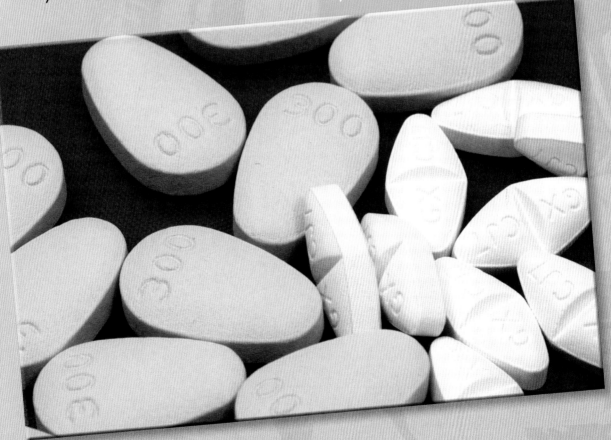

Tuberculosis

Tuberculosis has been around for thousands of years. It has had many names over the centuries, such as "white death," "consumption," and "the coughing plague." Today, the disease is usually simply called TB, and it is another major cause of death in some parts of the world.

What Causes TB?

TB is caused by a bacterium called *Mycobacterium tuberculosis*. When the bacterium is inhaled it infects the lungs, destroying tissue and gradually making breathing more difficult. If it is not treated, it spreads to other parts of the body, causing them to waste away. Eventually, the sufferer dies.

TB spreads when infected people cough and sneeze, so it can move from person to person quickly in crowded places, such as cities.

In the nineteenth century, when cities in Europe and the United States grew rapidly during the Industrial Revolution, TB was a major problem. At its height, TB caused one in every four deaths in New York City and London. As living standards improved, levels of TB in the developed world fell. From the 1940s onward, drugs were developed to treat it. Today, 85 percent of TB cases occur in the overcrowded countries of Africa and Asia, particularly India and China. There are about 9 million new cases every year, and 2 million deaths.

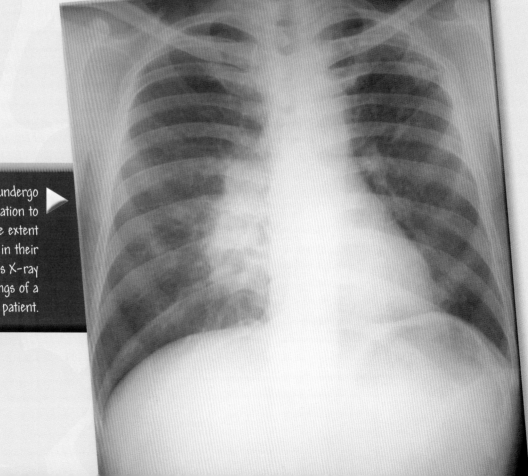

TB sufferers undergo X-ray examination to determine the extent of the infection in their lungs. This X-ray shows the lungs of a 49-year-old TB patient.

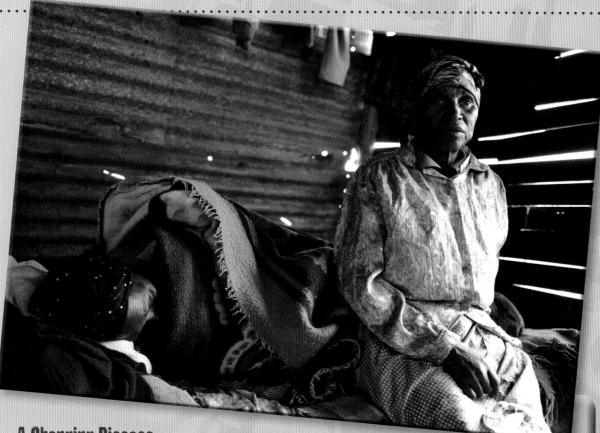

In a rural area of Natal in South Africa, a woman suffering from TB is cared for by a friend. She is also HIV-positive.

A Changing Disease

Like other infectious diseases, TB can change and become resistant to drug treatments, so the battle to defeat the disease is complex and difficult. A new strain of TB, multidrug-resistant TB, is the most challenging to treat. Furthermore, there is a strong link between TB and HIV, because TB thrives when the body's immune system is weak. About 10 percent of all TB cases are among people already living with HIV. Almost all these people are in Africa.

As so often is the case with disease, it is the poorest of the poor who are the worst hit by TB. Drug-resistant TB is also beginning to return to some large cities in the developed world, such as London and Paris, creating a new public health crisis.

COUNTDOWN!

The Stop TB Partnership, an organization formed in 2000 and committed to wiping out TB, estimates that this curable disease kills three people every minute. Without a rapid increase in efforts to treat and prevent TB, many millions more people will die from it in the future.

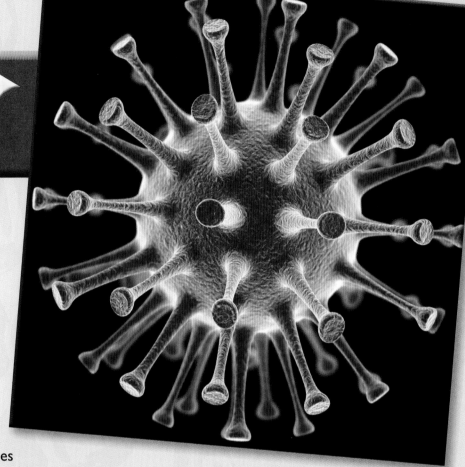

There are many types of flu viruses. This image shows a magnified version of just one strain.

Influenza

Influenza is most often simply called "the flu." A virus causes it, but there are many different types of flu viruses. This is one of the reasons why the illness is so difficult to control, and why flu epidemics regularly take hold around the world. Some of these epidemics have turned into devastating pandemics.

What Causes the Flu?

The flu generally attacks the body's respiratory system, including the lungs, the throat, and the nose. It brings fever, coughing, weakness, and sweating. It can affect anyone, of any age, although the very young and old are often most at risk. The flu spreads easily from person to person, carried through the air in water droplets when people sneeze, cough, or even laugh. The flu tends to peak in the winter in countries with a temperate, or not extreme, climate, because people's resistance is lowered in colder weather. Most people recover from the flu within about a week, but people with low resistance can develop serious infections such as pneumonia. Worldwide, between one-quarter of a million and half a million people die of the flu every year. About 36,000 of those are in the United States.

LOOK TO THE PAST

In 2009, a new flu pandemic swept around the world. This was swine flu, a new strain of the HINI virus that caused the devastating 1918–1920 pandemic. Swine flu, so called because the virus is carried by pigs, began in Mexico, and spread rapidly to the United States, Europe, and around the world. Most cases were mild, but about 18,000 people died. The authorities reacted quickly with public health information programs, and a vaccine was available within a few months.

Chasing the Virus

The three main groups of flu viruses are known as A, B, and C. The most common groups in humans are A and B, with A-group viruses causing the most severe disease. The A group of viruses often originates in wild birds, and spreads to other animals such as chickens and pigs. The viruses then pass from infected animals to the humans who handle them.

The most challenging aspect of the flu is that there are so many types of it, because the viruses can change so easily. Every few years the viruses make new strains to which people have no immunity. These cause new epidemics, or pandemics, that can affect millions of people.

Bird flu spreads from wild birds to farm birds such as chickens. People who handle the birds can then catch the virus.

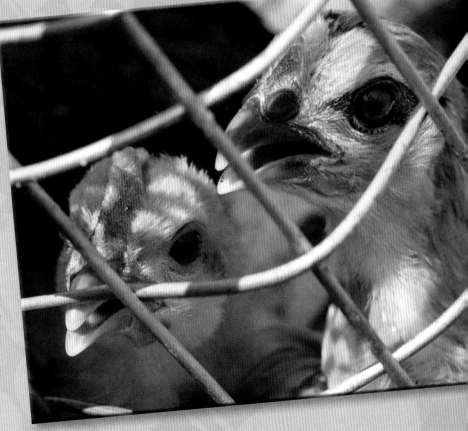

Cholera

Cholera is a disease that is carried in water. In the early nineteenth century, infected sailors and traders brought it from India to the West. It spread rapidly, causing several pandemics in Asia, Europe, and the Americas. Today, the disease is mostly confined to the developing world, where it is still a terrible threat to health.

In many underdeveloped countries, people use their drinking water supplies for washing and to also water their livestock. This can lead to outbreaks of diseases such as cholera.

What Causes Cholera?

Cholera is caused by a bacterium called *Vibrio cholerae*, which usually lives in standing water such as that used for drinking. When people swallow the water, the bacteria multiply inside their intestines and cause vomiting and severe diarrhea. Infected people can quickly become severely dehydrated, and without treatment they can die. In countries without advanced water and sewage treatment systems, the water supply can become contaminated with cholera. This also occurs after natural

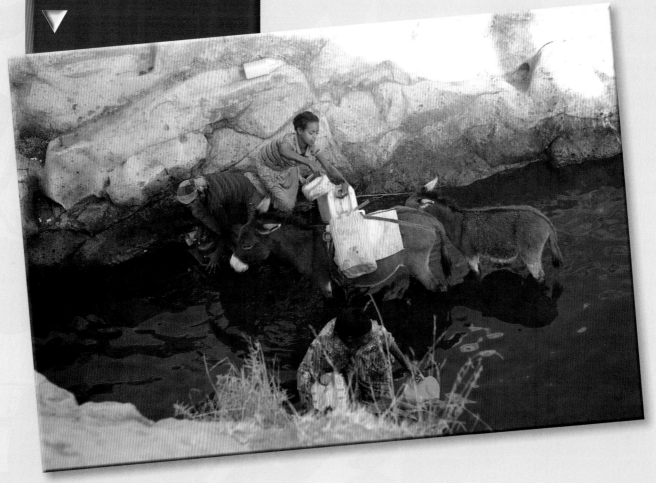

disasters, such as earthquakes and floods, when sewage full of cholera bacteria pollutes the water supply that people use for drinking and preparing food. In 2004, unusually heavy rainfall caused severe flooding in Bangladesh. Millions of people were threatened with water-borne diseases such as cholera when their drinking water was contaminated with raw sewage. Cholera affects about 3 million to 5 million people around the world, and causes more than 100,000 deaths, each year.

This is slum housing in India. In conditions such as this, where access to clean drinking water is limited, cases of cholera often occur.

Beating the Disease

Cholera is treatable. It can be cured with a mixture of antibiotics and rehydration therapy. Once cholera takes hold, it is essential to start treatment quickly. The difficulty lies in getting treatment to the remote and poor communities where people are most often infected. Also, once cholera has infected the water supply it is difficult to remove the disease and infection spreads rapidly through communities.

SCIENCE SOLUTIONS

Cholera Vaccine

There is a vaccine against cholera, but it does not provide protection for a very long period. In addition, there are challenges in getting the vaccine to the countries that need it most. It is too expensive for many of them, and health services in those countries may not be developed enough to distribute it. Work is under way to develop a more affordable and effective vaccine.

CHAPTER THREE

Treatment

The race to control epidemics and the spread of major diseases threatening the world needs a twofold approach: treat people who are already sick, and prevent people from contracting the diseases in the first place. Treatment is sometimes only a short-term solution. For example, drugs are developed to target the specific pathogens that cause disease, but they may not be effective over the long term. Patients still need treatment now, however, and research into new ways to help them recover is ongoing.

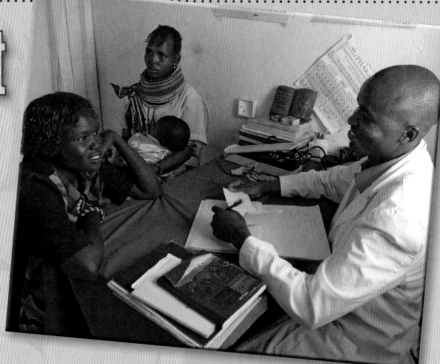

In Nairobi, Kenya, a doctor discusses treatment for HIV/AIDS with his patients in a clinic.

Simple Solutions

Sometimes treatment of disease can be remarkably simple. If, for instance, children are suffering from cholera, their most urgent need is to replace body salts and fluids lost through diarrhea. To achieve this, a simple and inexpensive packet of powdered medicine, containing sodium and potassium salts and sugar, can be dissolved in clean water and drunk. The children's rehydrated bodies are then much better able to fight off the infection. Millions of children's lives have been saved in this way.

Looking to Nature for Remedies

Other treatments can be found in nature. Until the development of modern medicine, plant remedies were the main form of treatment available for most diseases. Knowledge of plant medicine has been kept alive in some societies, and is still put to good use. The medicinal qualities of some plants have led to the development of drugs on a major scale. For example, the sweet wormwood plant was used in China for centuries to treat malaria. Scientists then identified the useful substances in the plant, and they have used them to develop the most effective antimalaria drugs in the world.

Learning from Experience

Doctors and other health professionals all over the world are engaged in the race to control epidemics. It is through years of experience in treating people that professionals learn which techniques and products work best. They can then build on that knowledge to create even better treatments for the future.

SCIENCE SOLUTIONS

Genetic Research

A key part of the treatment program for epidemic diseases is scientific research. For example, research into the genetic code of the bacteria or viruses that cause illness can help scientists understand exactly how diseases work. Knowing how diseases attack the immune system, or how they become resistant to some drugs, helps researchers design targeted treatments to defeat them.

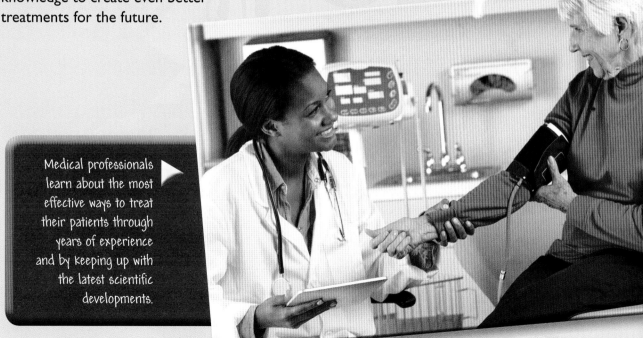

Medical professionals learn about the most effective ways to treat their patients through years of experience and by keeping up with the latest scientific developments.

Medication

The main weapon in the war against disease is medication. Some drugs have been in use for decades and are still effective. Others are being developed by the pharmaceutical industry all the time as people's knowledge of diseases improves. Once effective drugs have been developed, the next challenge is to get them to the people who need them most.

Attack from Different Directions

One common medicine used against infectious diseases is antibiotics. First developed in the mid-twentieth century to treat bacterial infections, antibiotics brought an immediate improvement to survival rates for diseases such as TB. Over time, however, the bacteria responsible for many diseases have evolved into new strains that are resistant to these drugs. New drugs must be developed all the time, to keep pace with changes in disease.

Viral infections, such as the flu, cannot be treated with antibiotics. If the disease is caught early enough, however, antiviral drugs can help. They make the symptoms of a disease less severe by preventing the virus from multiplying. If the virus has a strong hold on the body and has made it very weak, bacterial infections such as pneumonia can occur. These are treated with antibiotics.

Medication is at present the only treatment for the HIV virus. Patients take a large number of drugs every day, to slow the progress of HIV in the body and help prevent them from developing AIDS.

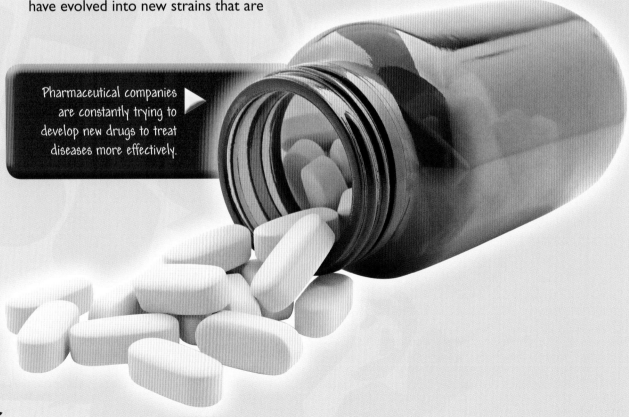

Pharmaceutical companies are constantly trying to develop new drugs to treat diseases more effectively.

Reaching the Poorest

Pharmaceutical research into drugs and their development can often take many scientists years of work. The drugs produced are therefore often expensive to buy. In developed countries with good health care systems, access to these drugs is relatively easy. In developing countries it is not.

Charitable organizations such as the Clinton Foundation—established by the former U.S. president Bill Clinton—are committed to improving this situation. They work with the pharmaceutical companies and the governments of developing countries to negotiate price reductions for drugs that target diseases such as malaria, TB, and HIV. They can also help to design products specifically for these poorer countries, and improve the chains of supply. It is estimated that drug-pricing agreements have saved the developing world more than $1 billion—and millions of lives.

President Bill Clinton (above) began the nonprofit Clinton Foundation to act as an intermediary between drug companies and the governments of developing countries. This and other organizations help make drugs for many serious diseases affordable and accessible.

COUNTDOWN!

Overuse of an antibiotic is the main reason it becomes ineffective. The more the bacteria are exposed to an antibiotic, the more likely they are to develop resistance to it. A new drug-resistant strain of TB is currently causing concern among health professionals.

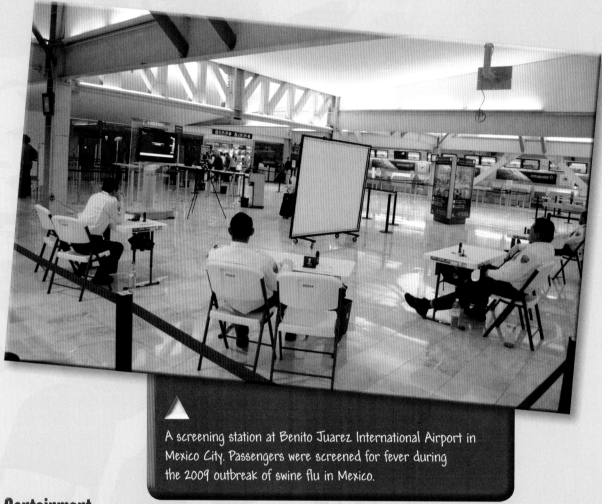

A screening station at Benito Juarez International Airport in Mexico City. Passengers were screened for fever during the 2009 outbreak of swine flu in Mexico.

Containment

When an epidemic begins, it is important to try to contain its spread. This means keeping infected people away from the rest of the population. It can also mean finding the source of the outbreak and removing that source. Often this is not possible. Some diseases arise in several places at once, and others, such as malaria, are already endemic in many countries.

Controlling the Spread

When a person becomes infected with the flu, he or she is advised to stay at home until all symptoms have passed. This is an effective way of controlling the spread of the disease —on a small scale. If levels of infection are high, and the disease is particularly serious, medical authorities may advise that public events be canceled. Infection can spread quickly at large-scale gatherings. People at increased risk, such as the elderly, may be advised to stay home.

Sometimes an epidemic is known to have originated in one country. This was the case with the swine flu epidemic of 2009, which started in Mexico. People leaving Mexico were screened for infection, and others were advised not to travel to the country.

Containing an Epidemic

The SARS epidemic of 2002–2003 began in China. This new disease, which originated in bats, caused severe breathing difficulties, diarrhea, and kidney failure. It affected around 8,000 people worldwide, about 700 of whom died. At the time, Asian nations imposed severe travel restrictions on anyone suspected of being infected with SARS. In China, anyone with symptoms was forced to spend one week in hospital, and was forbidden to see family members. These isolating measures helped to contain the epidemic.

LOOK TO THE PAST

In London, in 1853, cholera was killing hundreds of people in one overcrowded district. Its cause was still unknown, but one doctor, John Snow, noticed that the people affected were all obtaining their drinking water from one pump in the street. He removed the handle from the pump so it could not be used. The epidemic stopped three days later. This was a major breakthrough in the understanding of the disease.

During epidemic crises, health officials, such as the director of CDC, Dr. Thomas Frieden, update the press and public about the situation.

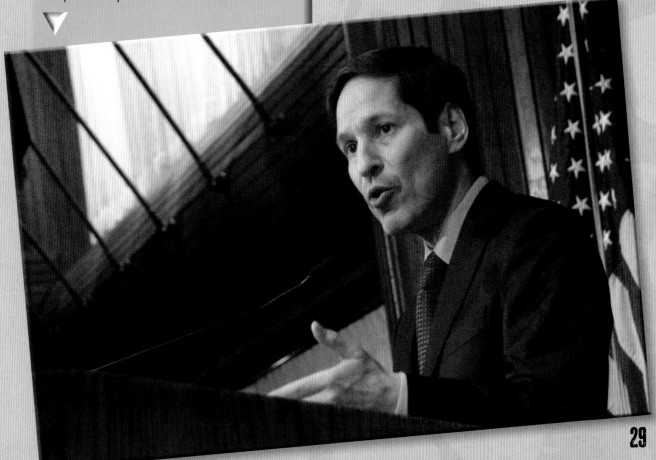

CHAPTER FOUR

Prevention

It is always better to prevent disease than it is to have to treat it. A large part of the race to control epidemics is focused on how to prevent them occurring in the first place. Some measures are quite simple, and relate to the ways people behave and look after themselves. Others are firmly rooted in cutting-edge science. Combined, all these measures are saving millions of lives around the world.

Becoming Immune to Disease

By far the most successful prevention measure in the fight to stop disease—and one of the great success stories of global health over the past 60 years or more—is immunization. This means giving people a vaccine, usually as an injection, against a specific disease, such as cholera or the flu. A vaccine is a weak dose of the disease, given in a form that will not make the person sick but will make his or her immune system respond by learning how to fight the disease with antibodies. If the person then later encounters the full disease, the immune system can recognize and destroy it.

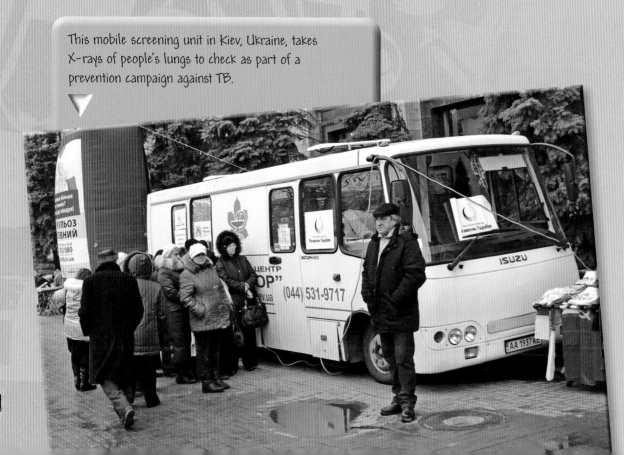

This mobile screening unit in Kiev, Ukraine, takes X-rays of people's lungs to check as part of a prevention campaign against TB.

SCIENCE SOLUTIONS

Rwanda

The results of malaria treatment and prevention measures speak for themselves. Between 2005 and 2007, after distributing insecticide-treated mosquito nets and providing sick patients with the right drug treatments, malaria deaths among young children in Rwanda, Africa, decreased by 66 percent.

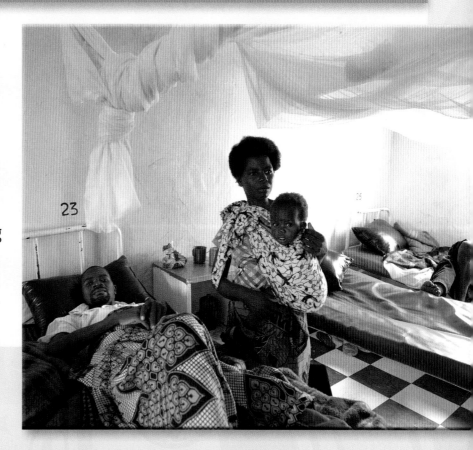

Simple But Effective

Other prevention measures are more straightforward, but no less important. One of the most successful weapons in the fight against malaria is a mosquito net treated with insecticide. The mosquitoes that carry malaria are most active at night, so people sleeping under treated nets have excellent protection against the insects. Hundreds of millions of nets have been distributed to countries affected by malaria, and this work is continuing. Other techniques include spraying the interiors of people's homes with insecticide to kill mosquitoes, and killing mosquitoes in their breeding grounds of still water.

Pregnant women have an increased risk of getting malaria and becoming very sick, and even dying. Giving women at least two doses of antimalarial drugs during their pregnancy has dramatically increased their chances of remaining healthy.

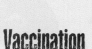

A child receives vaccination drops against polio, as part of a campaign to reduce levels of the disease in Pakistan.

Vaccination

The use of vaccination programs in both the developed and the developing world has had an enormous effect on controlling epidemics. Immunization is estimated to prevent the deaths of between 2 million and 3 million children each year. More than 1 million children, however, still die every year from diseases that could be prevented by vaccines.

Beating Measles

Many highly infectious diseases have been contained by immunization with vaccine. For example, measles is a serious viral disease that, in the worst cases, can be fatal. An effective vaccine was introduced in the developed world in the late 1960s, and a high percentage of the population in these countries was immunized. The number of deaths from the disease fell from 2.6 million in 1980 to 156,000 in 2012.

Vaccination rates in developing countries have improved greatly in recent years. By 2012, 84 percent of children globally received one dose of measles vaccine by their second birthday. The lowest figures are in Africa, with 73 percent of children, and Southeast Asia, with 78 percent, being immunized.

Chasing Flu Viruses

The flu is another epidemic disease that is controlled by vaccination. Every year, millions of people in the developed world get an annual flu shot. This can protect them against many of the most recent known strains of the illness. When new strains appear, scientists must develop new vaccines quickly. In some places in Asia, vaccination of chickens and other domesticated birds against bird flu has helped to prevent the spread of the disease. Sometimes it is necessary to destroy entire flocks of birds instead, in case they are infected.

Benefits of Research

Sometimes progress with one vaccine can help in the development of other vaccines. For example, if scientists discover a new ingredient that helps a vaccine to work well, or a new manufacturing process that makes it cheaper to produce, the whole field of vaccine research benefits.

LOOK TO THE PAST

For centuries, the lethal viral disease smallpox spread in epidemics around the world, killing millions. This was the first disease to be treated with vaccine. Thanks to a massive vaccination program, by the 1960s smallpox had disappeared from the developed world. WHO then coordinated another intensive smallpox vaccination program in the developing world. By 1979 it had been wiped out there, too. This encouraged global efforts to defeat more diseases in this way.

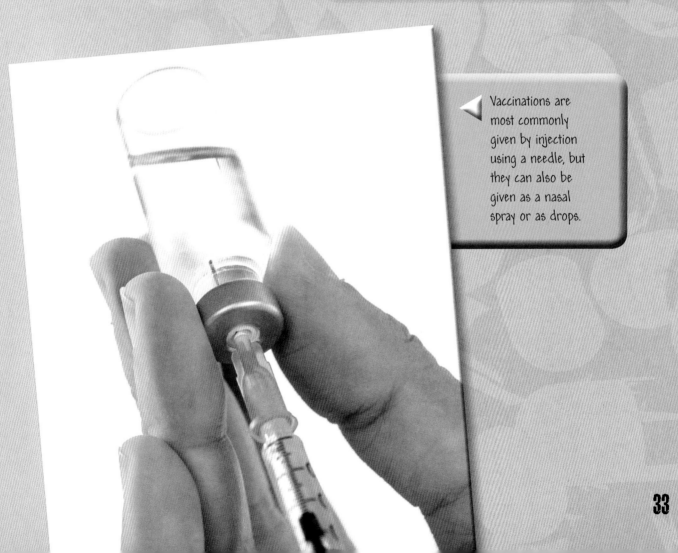

Vaccinations are most commonly given by injection using a needle, but they can also be given as a nasal spray or as drops.

Personal Behavior

Some of the tools ordinary people are using in the race to control epidemics are quite simple. Small changes in people's behavior can have an enormous impact on their chances of catching disease, or recovering if they become sick.

The children in this village have access to clean water from a properly installed pump. Having access to clean water is vital to teaching people the importance of good hygiene measures.

Keeping Healthy

Healthy people are less likely to get sick from many of the diseases that spread as epidemics. Fighting disease is all about keeping the body's immune system in good shape so the body can combat the disease-causing pathogens effectively. A healthy lifestyle helps keep the immune system working well. This includes a good diet, with plenty of fruits and vegetables, and not too many fatty or sugary foods. Fruit and vegetables give the body the vitamins and minerals it needs. Maintaining a healthy immune system also includes getting plenty of exercise and sleep, to allow the body to repair itself.

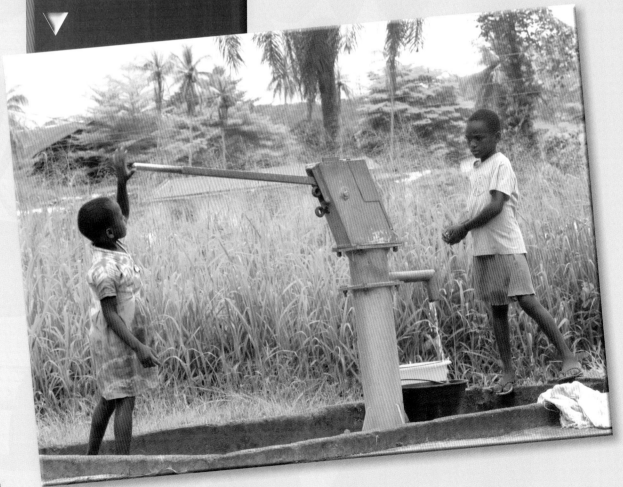

Soap and Water

Hygiene is another important aspect of disease prevention. The simple act of washing one's hands remains one of the most important things that can be done to protect people from disease. It seems amazing that even deadly bacteria and viruses can be killed by soap. Washing with soap for at least 20 seconds removes most of the pathogens on the skin, and so reduces the chance of them getting into the body. People should wash with soap after preparing food, using the toilet, and being in public places.

However, a few viruses cannot be removed by washing alone. Some strains of the norovirus, for example, which regularly cause outbreaks of vomiting and diarrhea, are very hard to remove completely by washing.

In developing countries, people may have to walk miles every day to find a water source, which may be polluted. Giving those people easy access to clean water and good sanitation facilities can make a big difference to the spread of diseases such as cholera and typhoid.

SCIENCE SOLUTIONS

Soap removes the germs from our hands when we wash them, not the hot water. The water from our faucets is unlikely to be hot enough to kill germs, which are attached to the oily surface of our skin. The soap detaches this oily coating from our hands, and lifts the germs away with it. We need water to wash the germ-covered soap away, but it does not have to be very hot to do this effectively.

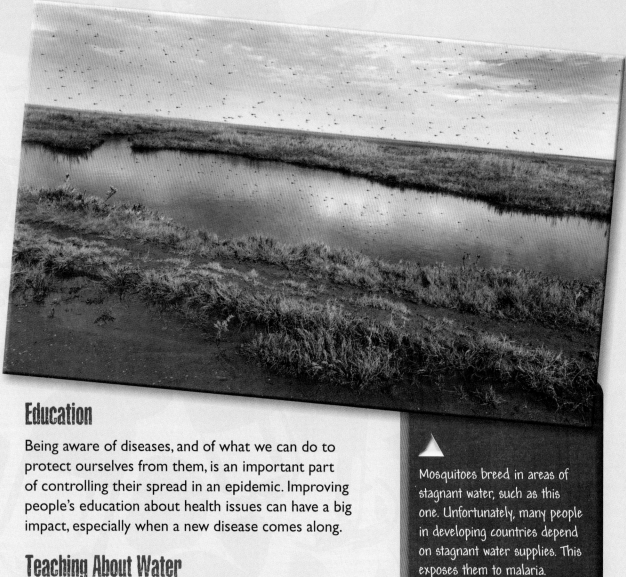

Education

Being aware of diseases, and of what we can do to protect ourselves from them, is an important part of controlling their spread in an epidemic. Improving people's education about health issues can have a big impact, especially when a new disease comes along.

Teaching About Water

In countries with a malaria problem, education programs teach people about the dangers of stagnant water, where mosquitoes breed. Programs also teach about the importance of good hygiene and sanitation in the fight against many infectious diseases, but especially cholera and typhoid, which are carried in polluted water. Having a standpipe to supply clean water and a series of properly-built latrines, or outdoor toilets, can make an enormous difference to people's health.

Mosquitoes breed in areas of stagnant water, such as this one. Unfortunately, many people in developing countries depend on stagnant water supplies. This exposes them to malaria.

A Worldwide Battle

One of the most successful awareness campaigns in the developed world took place in the 1980s and 1990s, when HIV/AIDS first appeared. Advertisements in the media, many of which were hard-hitting, warned people of the dangers of the disease and explained how they could protect themselves against it. This had a major impact on people's behavior in an attempt to control the spread of the disease.

Unfortunately, HIV/AIDS has now become a pandemic in the developing world. There, huge effort is being put into education and awareness campaigns to try to control the spread of the disease.

December 1 is World AIDS Day. This event is designed to increase awareness and improve education about the disease all over the world. It also reminds governments of the need to continue the fight against HIV/AIDS by investing and supporting new technologies.

COUNTDOWN!

Globally, 34 million people have HIV/AIDS. About 1 million of those are in the United States. Since 1981, more than 25 million people have died from AIDS. This makes it one of the most destructive pandemics in history.

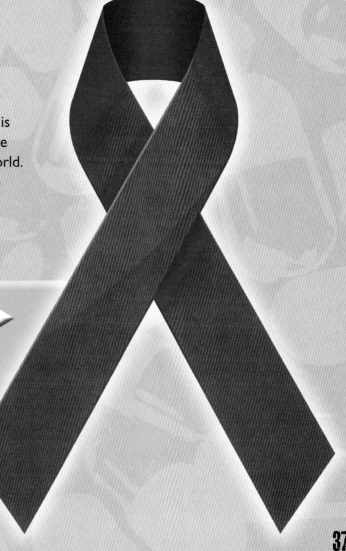

On World AIDS Day millions of people buy and wear a red ribbon as a sign of their support for the fight against the disease.

CHAPTER FIVE

The Future

The fight against epidemics is being fought on many fronts. All over the world people are working on treatment and prevention methods that may stop the spread of the worst diseases. Some people are dealing with immediate crises while others are working on long-term solutions.

Getting Vaccines to the People

One priority for the future is to increase rates of vaccination in the developing world. WHO estimates that two-thirds of the preventable deaths among children in the developing world are from pneumonia and the rotavirus, which causes severe diarrhea. There are vaccines for both these diseases. By 2015, the health organization Global Alliance for Vaccines and Immunization (GAVI) plans to introduce rotavirus vaccines to 30 of the world's poorest countries, and pneumonia vaccines to 45 developing countries.

Global Action

The Stop TB Partnership is a global movement of more than 1,200 organizations that aims to eliminate TB around the world. The movement's achievements are impressive. Infection and death rates from TB are declining, but there is still a long way to go.

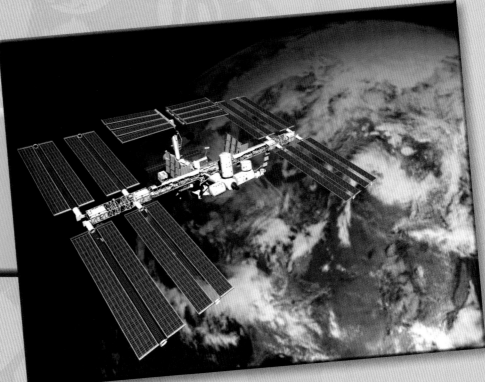

Satellites in space can be used to help track and predict patterns in the spread of diseases, for example by looking at currents in the oceans.

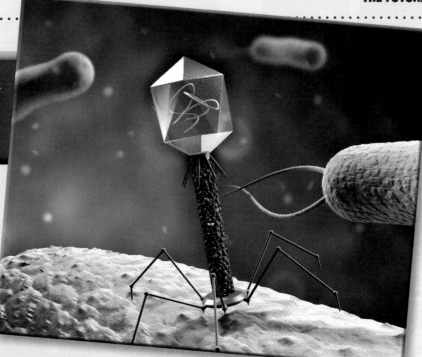

This is an artist's impression of a bacteriophage attacking bacteria.

A similar partnership, Roll Back Malaria, is coordinating global action against malaria. Its 500 partners are working together on prevention and treatment measures, and the results have been outstanding. Eight countries in Africa, including Botswana, Namibia, and Rwanda, have reduced their levels of malaria by more than 50 percent since 2000.

Early Epidemic Warnings

Another key area of research is the prediction of disease patterns. This means looking at data on topics such as changes in climate or the movement of people. For example, cholera outbreaks have been found to follow seasonal increases in sea temperature. Satellites in space can now look at ocean current movements and predict temperature increases well in advance, providing an early-warning system for countries such as India and Bangladesh, where cholera epidemics are frequent.

SCIENCE SOLUTIONS

Bacteriophages

Scientists have found a new way to make vaccines that could be very useful in developing countries. Some viruses, called bacteriophages, kill bacteria. They can be given to humans to vaccinate them against bacterial infections. Like all viruses, they multiply extremely quickly, so they are simple and cheap to produce. It should even be possible to protect against several bacteria with just a single bacteriophage shot. Bacteriophages could also treat bacterial infections that have become resistant to antibiotics.

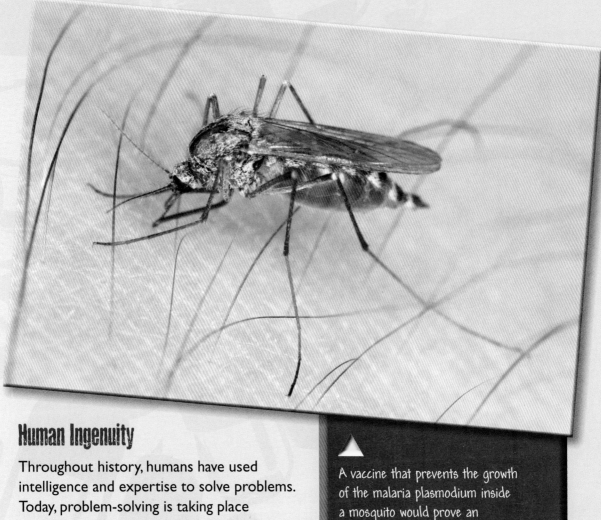

A vaccine that prevents the growth of the malaria plasmodium inside a mosquito would prove an ingenious solution to malaria.

Human Ingenuity

Throughout history, humans have used intelligence and expertise to solve problems. Today, problem-solving is taking place on a huge scale as new technologies are developed to improve the supply of disease-fighting weapons.

Ingenious Malaria Prevention

At present there is no vaccine for malaria, but clever solutions are being tested. There are potential new malaria vaccines that are designed to block the growth of the malaria plasmodium within the mosquito itself. The infected mosquito bites a vaccinated human and sucks up his or her blood. In this blood the mosquito receives a dose of the vaccine and this prevents it from passing on the plasmodium to another human.

This has become possible only because scientists have figured out the genetic make-up of the malaria plasmodium.

TB and AIDS Research

The search for new TB vaccines is also under way. TB is a major cause of death among people with HIV/AIDS, so research into the two diseases is closely linked. In a recent breakthrough, researchers discovered some powerful antibodies that seem to be able to destroy the

HIV virus in the body. This had not been possible before because the HIV virus had always changed to avoid the effects of vaccines. The antibodies will now be tested, and could form a vital part of treatment in the future.

Quick Wins

It takes years to develop new vaccines, and it costs millions of dollars. However, sometimes progress can come in a simpler form. Medical professionals need to diagnose disease quickly, so they can provide the correct treatment and limit the spread of infection. New rapid diagnostic tests (RDTs) for malaria have enabled medics in poor and remote areas to diagnose malaria from just a small sample of the patient's blood, without the need for expensive equipment. If the malaria test proves positive, treatment can begin without delay. If not, expensive drugs need not be wasted.

SCIENCE SOLUTIONS

Universal Flu Vaccine

Flu vaccines are made available every year, but they can only respond to known strains of the disease. Scientists are now working on a universal flu vaccine, meaning it works on all strains. If scientists can identify and target the parts of the flu virus that do not change from one strain to another, they could revolutionize the vaccination effort. It is only a matter of time before the next flu pandemic occurs.

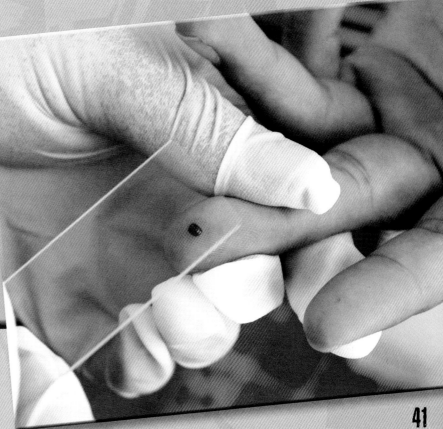

New simple tests that can be used in resource-poor areas are making a big difference to the diagnosis and treatment of diseases such as malaria.

The Bigger Picture

Epidemics are closely linked to even bigger issues facing the world today: poverty and inequality. These issues cause many of the situations that dramatically worsen the outbreak and spread of disease.

Odds Stacked Against the Poor

The flu and other epidemics can affect any part of the world. However, the overwhelming majority of epidemics occur in the world's poorest countries. Malaria, TB, cholera, and HIV are big problems in the developing world. The race to control them, therefore, includes measures to improve the living standards of people in these countries.

People's immune systems are weakened when they do not have enough to eat, or they have to work constantly just to survive. In big cities, overcrowding and poor sanitation make outbreaks of infectious diseases such as cholera and typhoid much more likely to occur. In rural areas, preventable and curable diseases such as malaria take hold when people are unaware of what is causing them. Health systems are poorly developed in many places, so that people cannot get access to medical care. Even when drugs and other treatments can be distributed, they are often too expensive for people to buy.

These people in Mozambique are searching for food in a landfill site. Living in such poverty exposes people to disease.

Global Steps Toward Improvement

Solving the problems of poverty and inequality is complicated, but an enormous amount is being done to tackle these issues. For example, governments and agencies around the world are investing in measures to improve educational opportunities that help people find jobs and grow enough food to feed themselves and their families. Standards of hygiene and sanitation are slowly improving in many places, as is access to medical care. All of these measures mean that when disease strikes, people are in a stronger position to fight back.

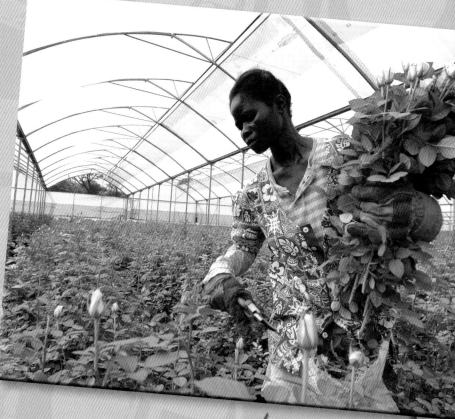

This woman in Zambia is employed in a business that exports flowers to Europe. Jobs such as these improve people's living standards.

COUNTDOWN!

The biggest cause of death among children younger than one year old is diarrhea caused by infection. This number is highest in developing countries, but they are getting smaller. In African countries south of the Sahara desert, the number of deaths per thousand births has fallen from 106 in 1990 to 63 in 2012, a reduction of approximately 40 percent. In South Asia, the reduction has been 49 percent in the same period.

Can We Win the Race?

People all over the world are committed to fighting epidemics. Some of them work in laboratories, researching vaccines, drugs, and medical techniques. Some work in governments and positions of authority, where their influence can make change happen. Others are working on the ground, helping people in the community. They may be health professionals, educators, or charity workers.

Real change can happen when there is genuine cooperation between people. For example, since 2000, global deaths from malaria have fallen by more than 26 percent. More than 1 million children's lives have been saved in Africa. Twenty-five countries are currently on track to eliminate malaria altogether in the not too distant future. This has been possible because of an increase in international funding for the fight against malaria.

The situation also looks good for other diseases. Prevention efforts have reduced the level of new cases of HIV in a growing number of countries, and the number of people receiving treatment for HIV/AIDS in developing countries has increased tenfold since 2000. The incidence of TB worldwide

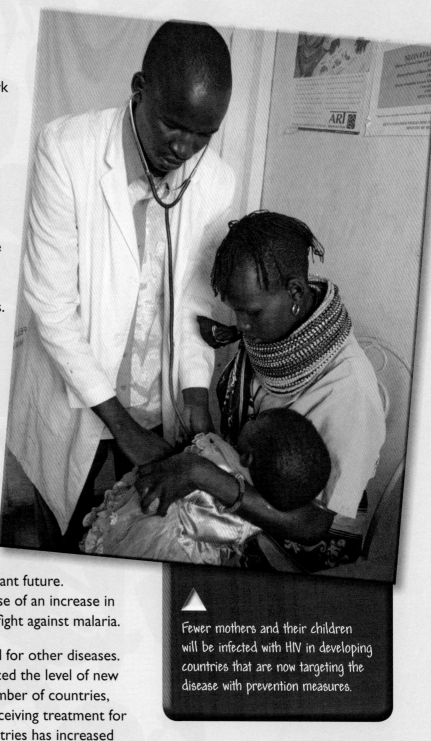

Fewer mothers and their children will be infected with HIV in developing countries that are now targeting the disease with prevention measures.

is also falling, but the new drug-resistant strains of the disease mean that efforts to find a vaccine still have a long way to go.

Finding the Cure

The widespread use of antibiotics, antivirals, and vaccines has dramatically reduced the death toll from epidemic diseases. Improved methods of diagnosis also ensure that patients get the correct treatment and get it quickly. There will always be new strains of disease that threaten us, but we are well-positioned to fight back.

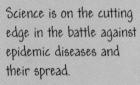

Science is on the cutting edge in the battle against epidemic diseases and their spread.

SCIENCE SOLUTIONS

Nanopatch Vaccine

Scientists are working on an exciting new way to give vaccines—the nanopatch. This small patch, coated in vaccine, is simply placed on a person's skin. Thousands of tiny projections on the patch then deliver the vaccine straight into cells just under the skin's surface. Skin cells seem to take up the vaccine even better than muscle cells, which is where vaccines are usually injected with a needle. The patch better suits remote, poor locations because unlike with traditional vaccines, its dose does not have to be kept refrigerated, and there are no needles to keep sterile. Also, a vaccine that now costs $10 if injected via a needle could cost just 10 cents if given through the nanopatch. This would greatly increase the number of people that developing countries could afford to vaccinate.

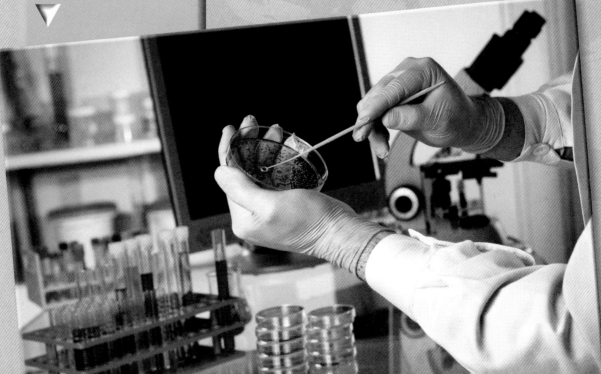

Glossary

antibiotic A drug that is used to kill bacteria that cause diseases.

antiviral A drug that is used to halt the development of viruses in the body.

bacteria Single-celled living pathogens that can cause disease.

bacteriophage A virus that kills bacteria.

cholera A bacterial disease, carried in polluted water and food, which causes severe diarrhea.

contaminated Made unclean or dangerous by a substance.

dehydrated To be severely lacking in water.

diagnosis To establish that a person has an illness or a disease.

endemic A situation where an infectious disease remains in the population and infects many people at any one time.

fatal Resulting in death.

HIV A virus that attacks the body's immune system and can lead to AIDS.

hygiene Cleanliness and good sanitation.

immunity Protection from a disease.

immunization The process of protecting people against harmful infections before they come into contact with them. This is usually done by injecting a vaccine.

immunodeficiency A situation where the body's immune system cannot fight disease effectively.

innovative Smart, a revolutionary new way of doing something.

insecticide A chemical mixture that kills insects.

malaria A disease caused by a protozoa carried by mosquitoes.

nanopatch A small patch that delivers vaccine into the skin.

pandemic An epidemic that has spread worldwide.

pathogen A microorganism that causes disease.

protozoa Single-celled living pathogens that can cause disease.

resistant Able to resist or withstand something.

sanitation Cleanliness in order to avoid illness or disease.

severity A degree of harshness.

vaccination The process where the body is given a weakened version of a disease so that the immune system can build up resistance to it.

virus A nonliving microorganism that causes disease when it invades the body.

Further Reading

Books

Bailey, Diane. *Cholera.* New York, NY: Rosen Publishing, 2011.

Ballard, Carol. *AIDS and Other Epidemics* (What If We Do Nothing?). New York, NY: Gareth Stevens, 2009.

Pendercrast, Mark. *Inside the Outbreaks: The Elite Medical Detectives of the Epidemic Intelligence Service.* New York, NY: Houghton Mifflin Harcourt, 2010.

Person, Stephen. *Malaria, Super Killer!* (Nightmare Plagues). New York, NY: Bearport Publishing, 2010.

Stille, Darlene R. *Outbreak! The Science of Pandemics* (Headline Science). Mankato, MN: Compass Point Books, 2010.

Web Sites

Due to the changing nature of Internet links, Rosen Publishing has developed an online list of Web sites related to the subject of this book. This site is updated regularly. Please use this link to access the list:

http://www.rosenlinks.com

Index